THE PICTURE BOOK OF

AMERICAN PATRIOTISM

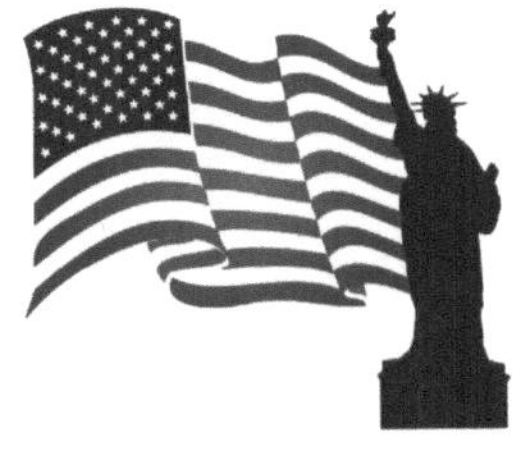

SUNNY STREET
BOOKS

Copyright © 2019 Sunny Street Books
All rights reserved.

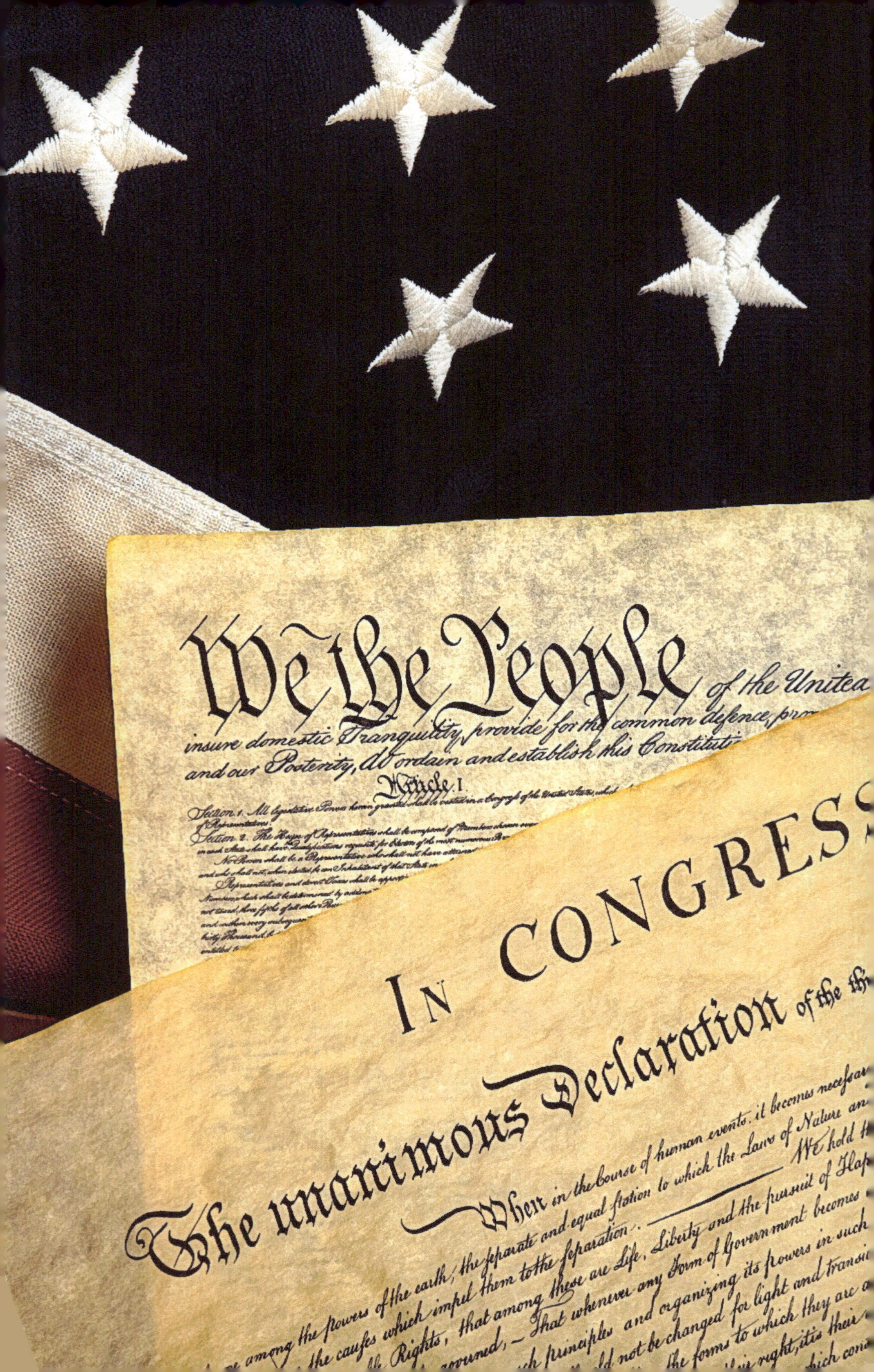
We the People of the United
insure domestic Tranquility, provide for the common defence,
and our Posterity, do ordain and establish this Constitut
Article. I.
In CONGRESS
The unanimous Declaration of the th
When in the Course of human events, it becomes necessar
the causes which impel them to the separation.
Rights, that among these are Life, Liberty and the pursuit of Happ
governed, — That whenever any Form of Government becomes

THE DECLARATION OF INDEPENDENCE

The Declaration of Independence was written during the American Revolution. It stated America's intention to be free of British rule. The Continental Congress formally adopted the Declaration of Independence in Philadelphia on July 4, 1776.

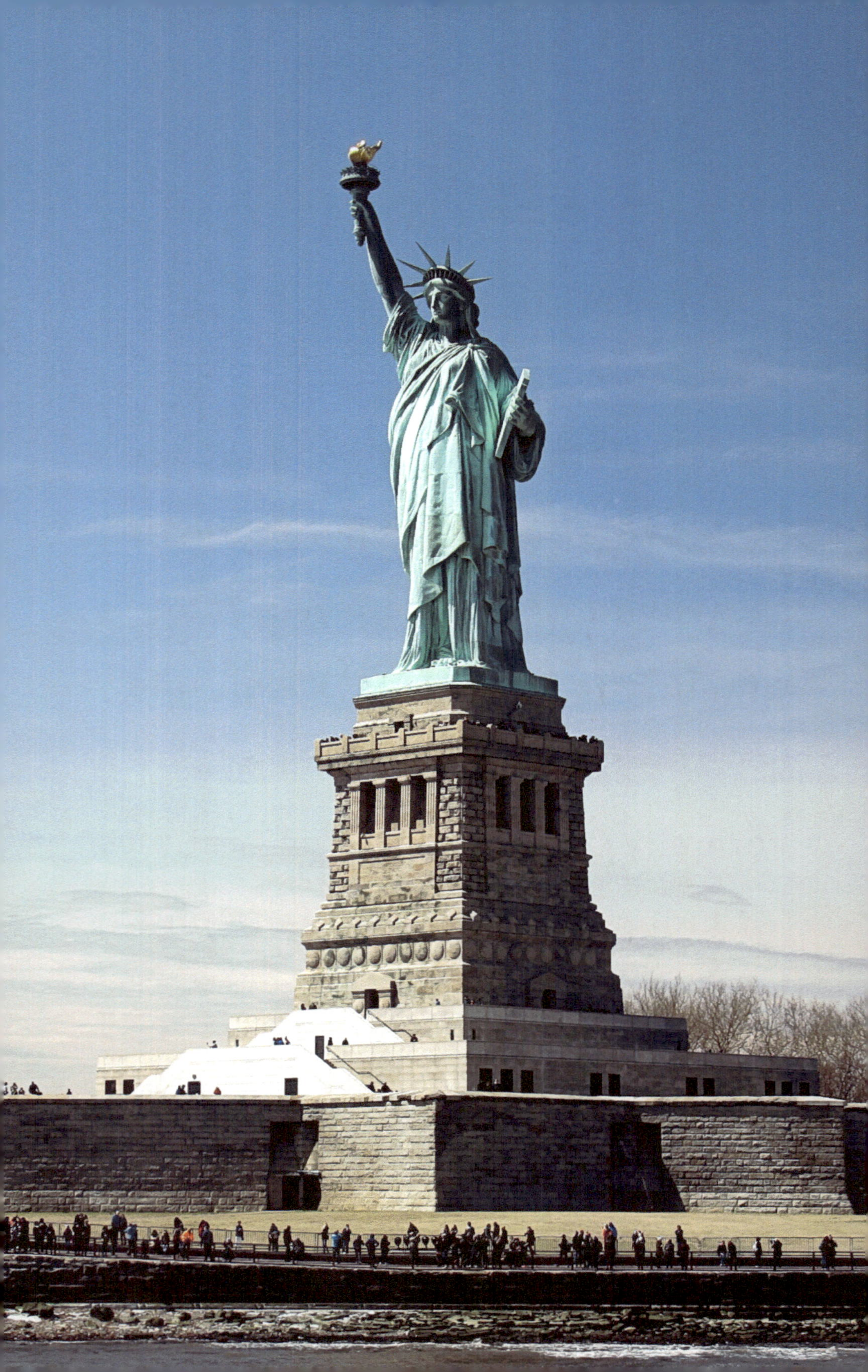

THE STATUE
OF LIBERTY

The Statue of Liberty was a gift of friendship from the people of France to the United States. It stands on Liberty Island in New York Harbor and is recognized as a universal symbol of freedom and democracy.

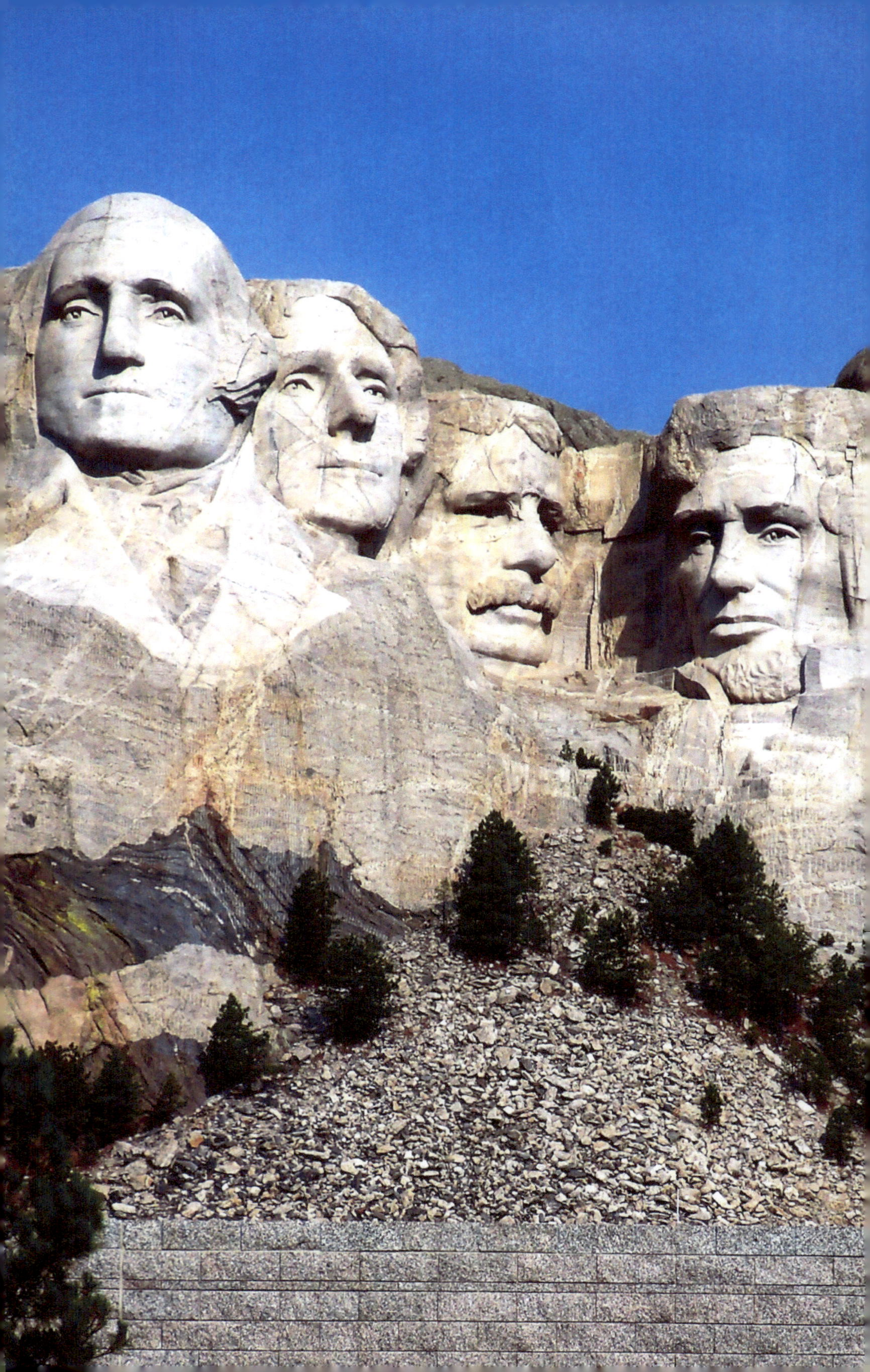

MOUNT RUSHMORE

Mount Rushmore is located in the Black Hills of South Dakota. It shows the faces of four American presidents: George Washington, Thomas Jefferson Theodore Roosevelt, and Abraham Lincoln. It took 14 years to carve at a cost of almost one million dollars.

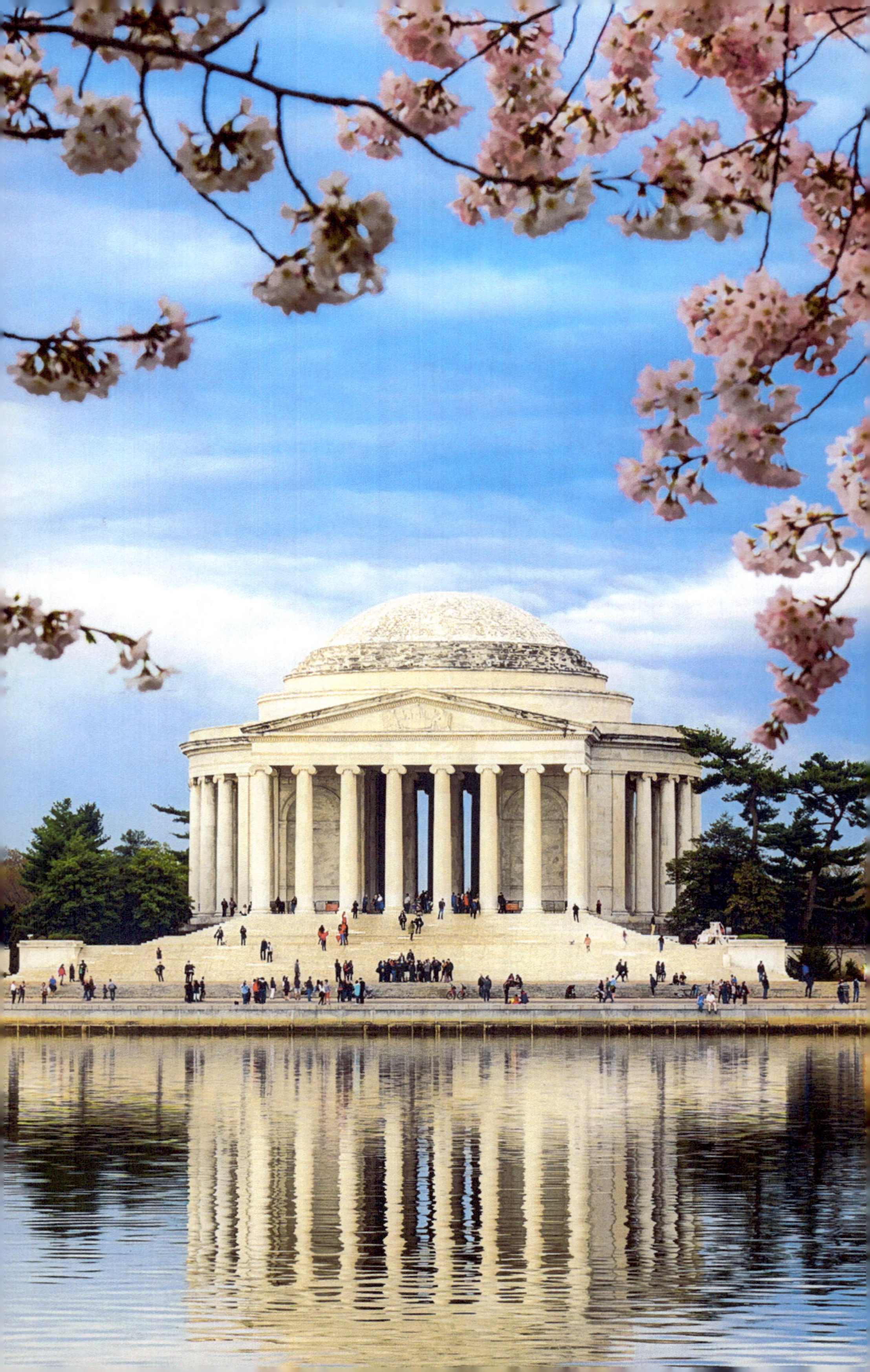

THE JEFFERSON MEMORIAL

This monument was built in honor of Thomas Jefferson, who was one of America's Founding Fathers. He was the main author of the Declaration of Independence, and later he served as the third president of the United States.

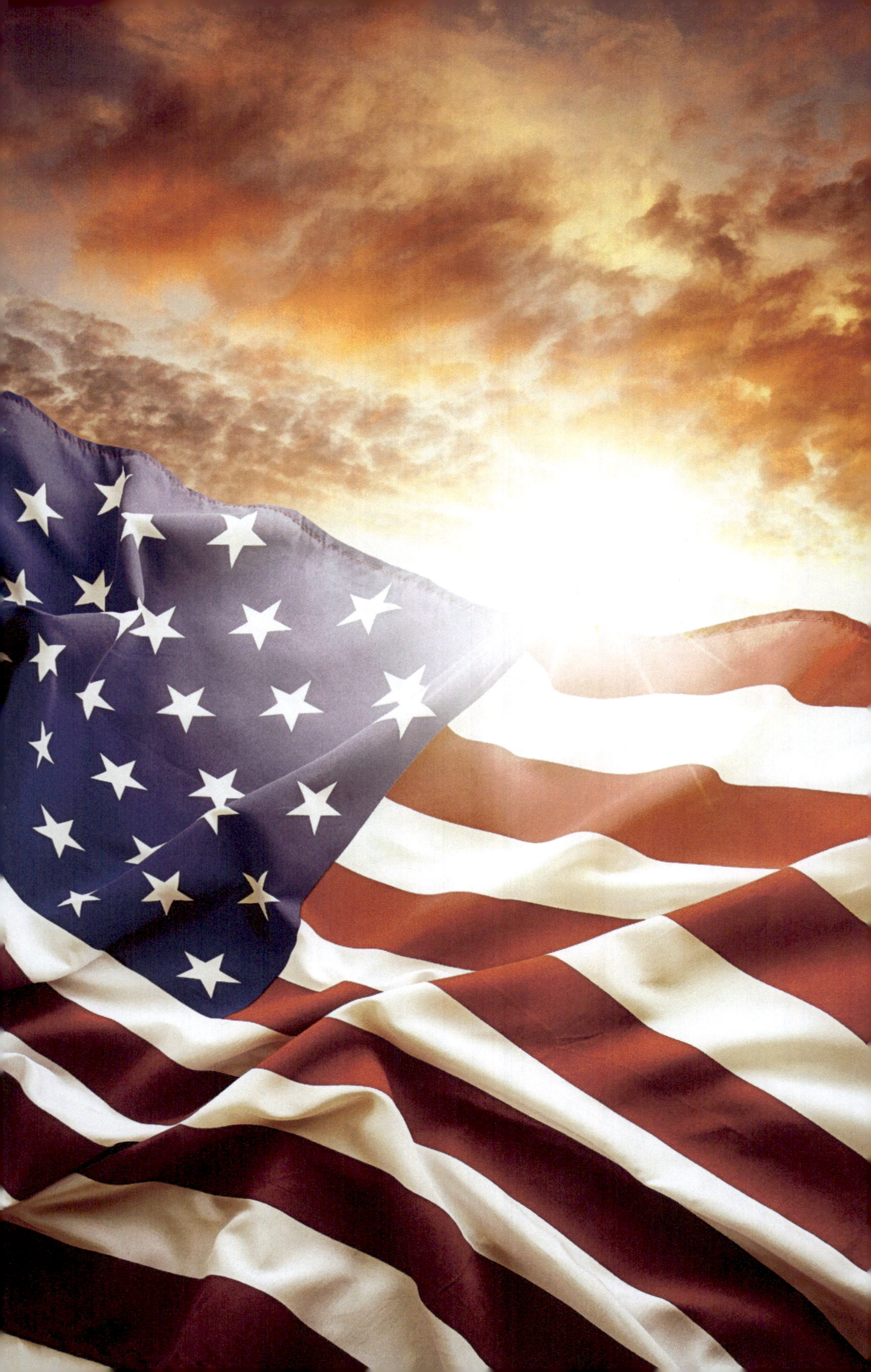

THE STAR SPANGLED BANNER

During the War of 1812, when Francis Scott Key realized the Americans had won the Battle of Baltimore over the British, he wrote a poem about the victory. It was later set to music and became "The Star Spangled Banner," which was adoped as our national anthem.

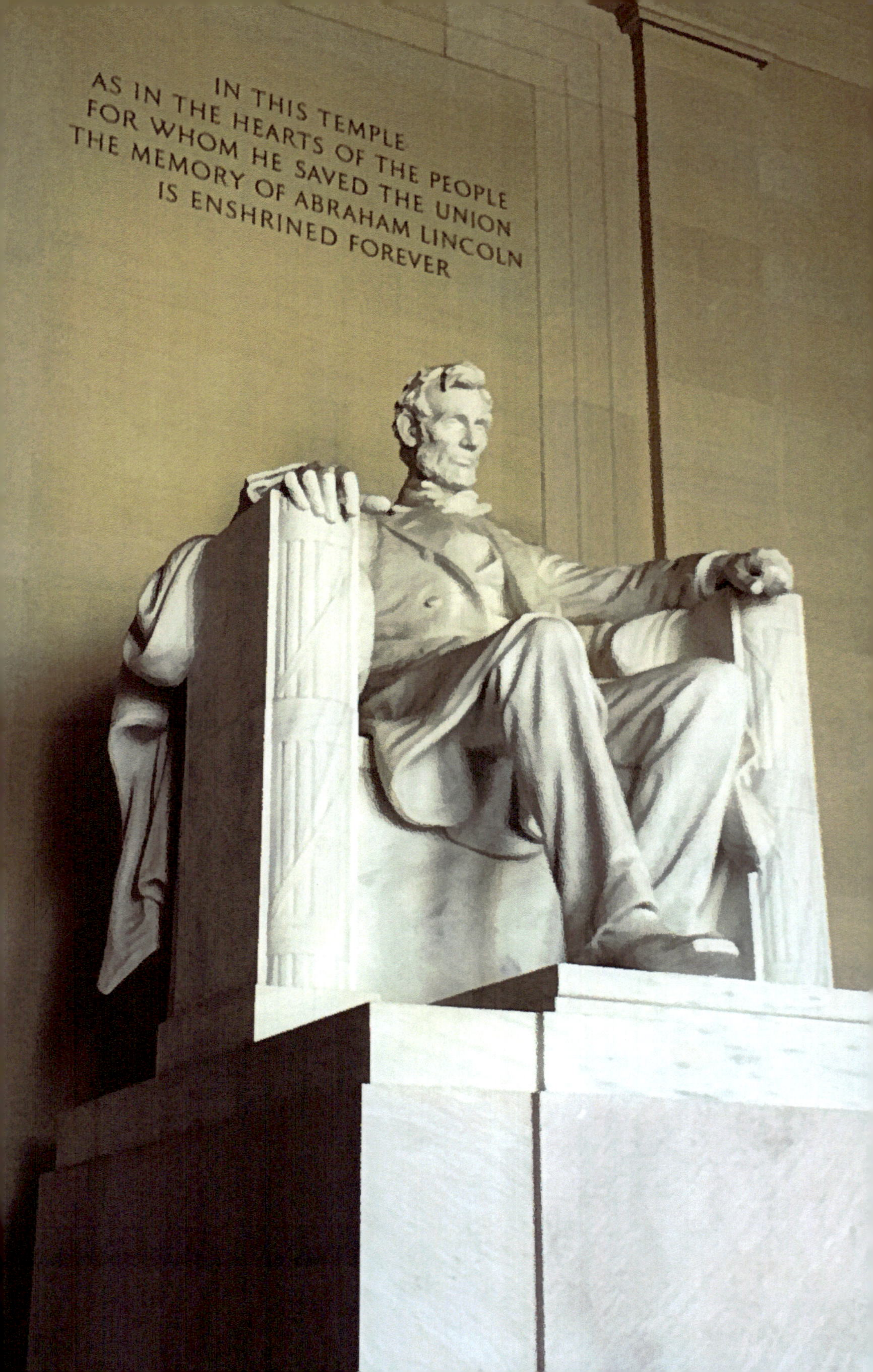

IN THIS TEMPLE
AS IN THE HEARTS OF THE PEOPLE
FOR WHOM HE SAVED THE UNION
THE MEMORY OF ABRAHAM LINCOLN
IS ENSHRINED FOREVER

THE LINCOLN MEMORIAL

The Lincoln Memorial is a monument in Washington, D.C that honors Abraham Lincoln, the 16th president of the United States. Its inscription reads, "In this temple, as in the hearts of the people for whom he saved the union, the memory of Abraham Lincoln is enshrined forever."

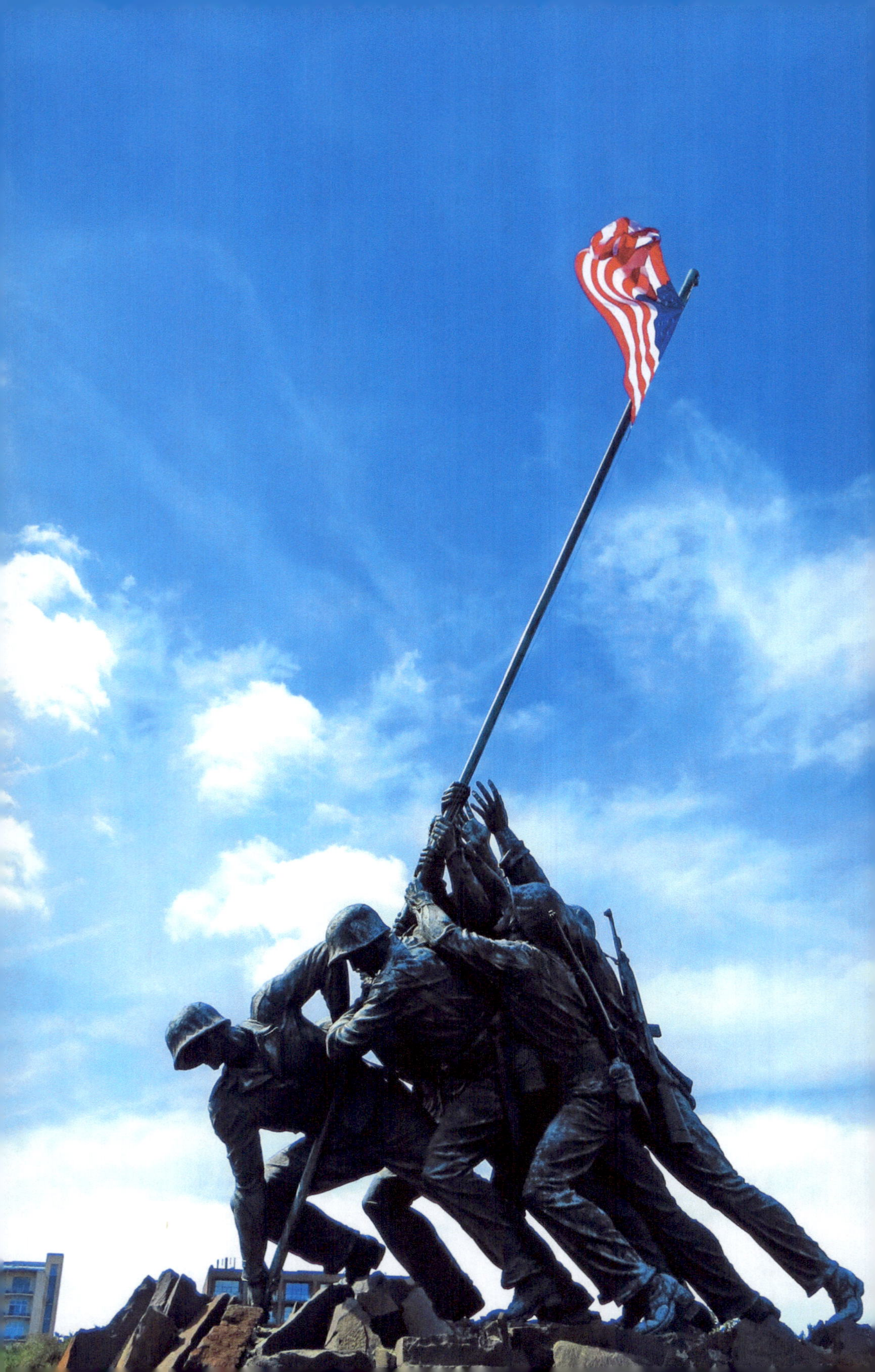

THE IWO JIMA MEMORIAL

This statue depicts one of the most famous photographs in history. It shows six brave men raising the American flag on the island of Iwo Jima, Japan during World War II.

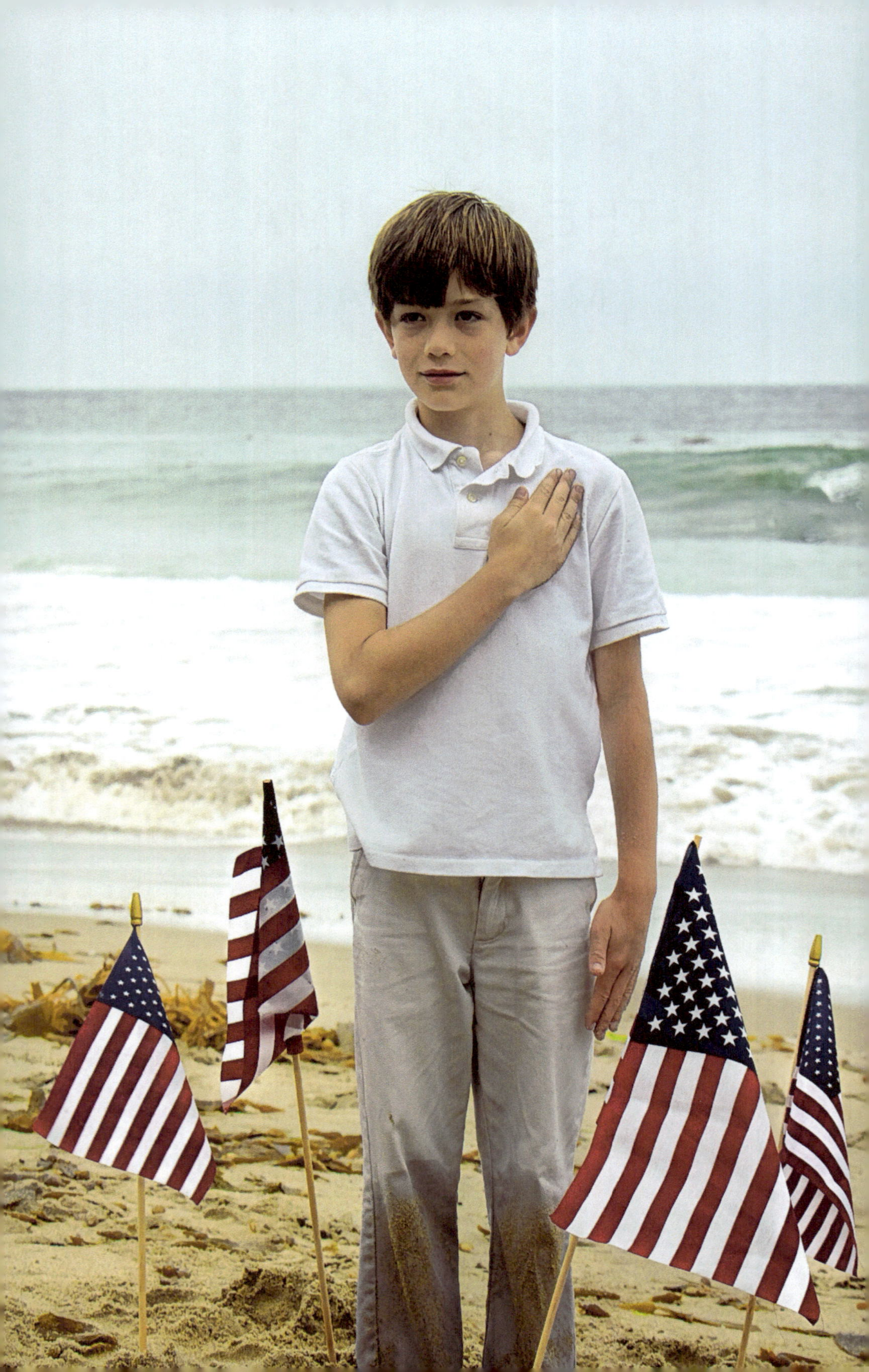

THE PLEDGE OF ALLEGIANCE

"I pledge allegiance to the flag of the United States of America, and to the republic for which it stands, one nation, under God, indivisible, with liberty and justice for all."

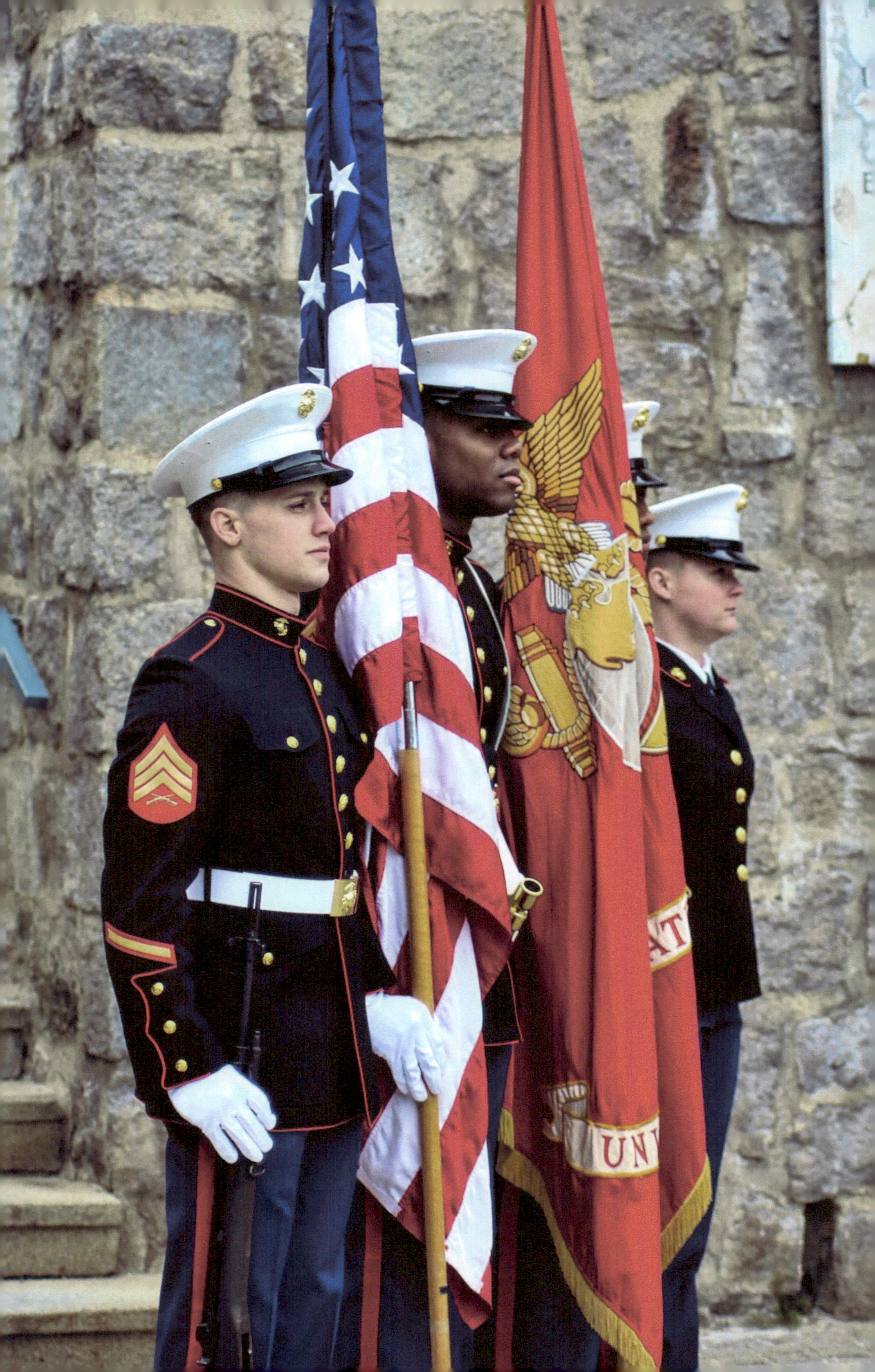

COLOR GUARD

A military Color Guard is a uniformed team of at least four active duty, reserve, or retired soldiers. It is their job to present and protect the flag of the United States, the flag of their branch of service, and various others. They perform at both military and civilian events.

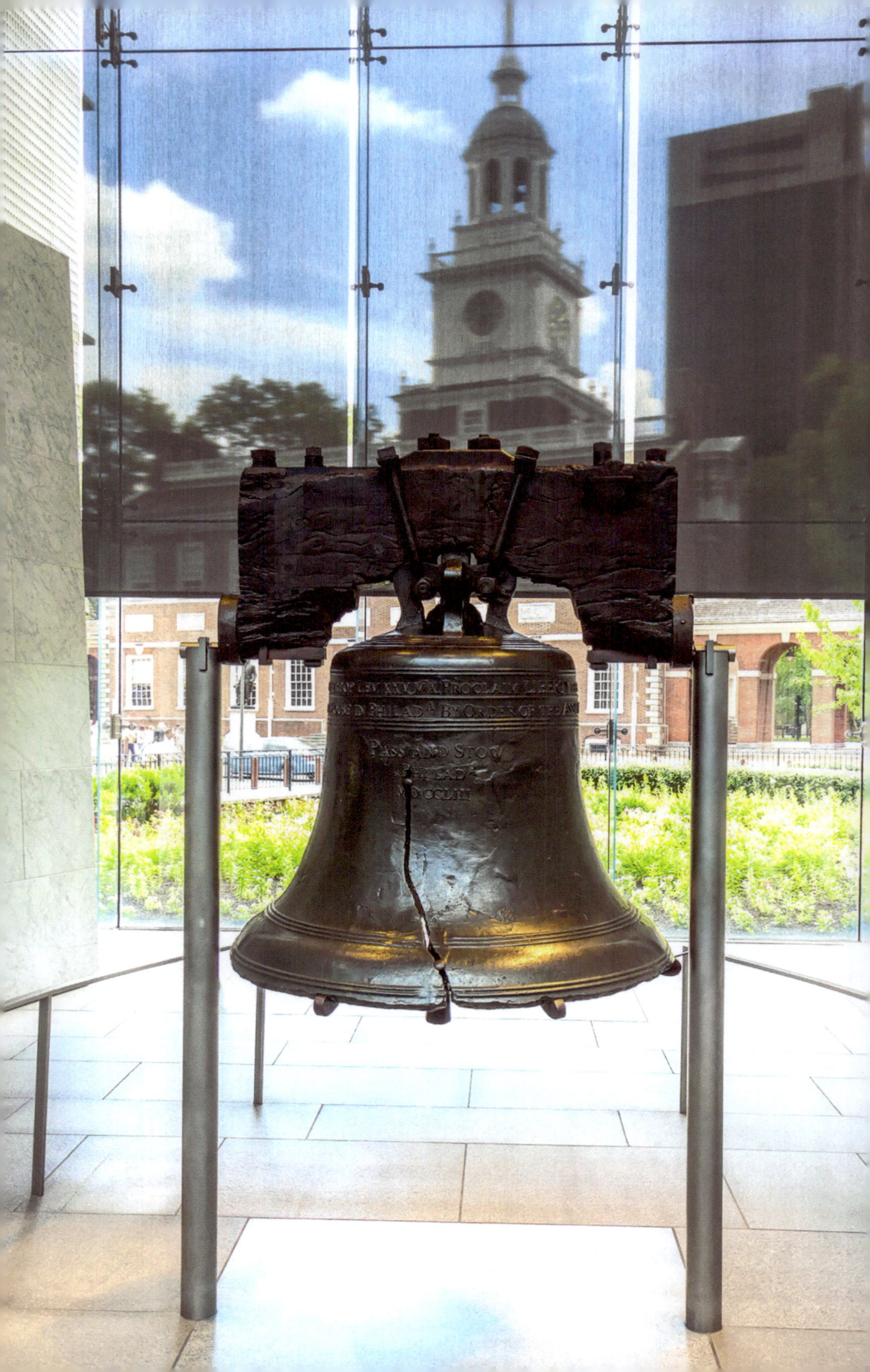
PROCLAIM LIBERTY
PASS AND STOW
PHILAD
MDCCLIII

THE LIBERTY BELL

Liberty Bell is a traditional symbol of American freedom. It was created in 1751 to hang in Philadelphia's Independence Hall. It was rung for the last time on George Washington's birthday in 1846, at which time it cracked and could not be fixed.

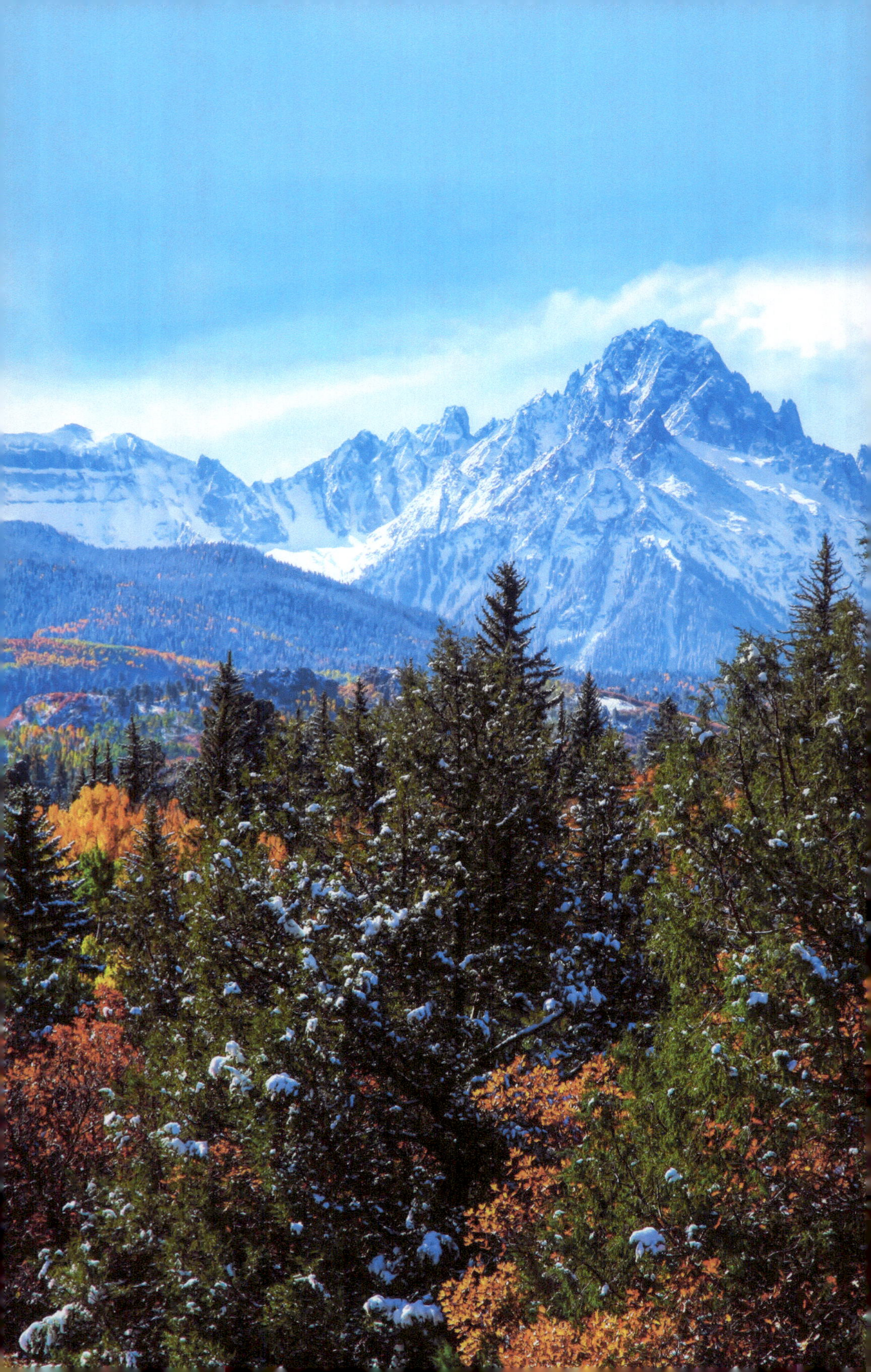

AMERICA
THE BEAUTIFUL

♪ Oh beautiful for spacious skies,

For amber waves of grain,

For purple mountain majesties

Above the fruited plain.

America! America!

God shed his grace on thee,

And crown thy good with

brotherhood

From sea to shining sea!

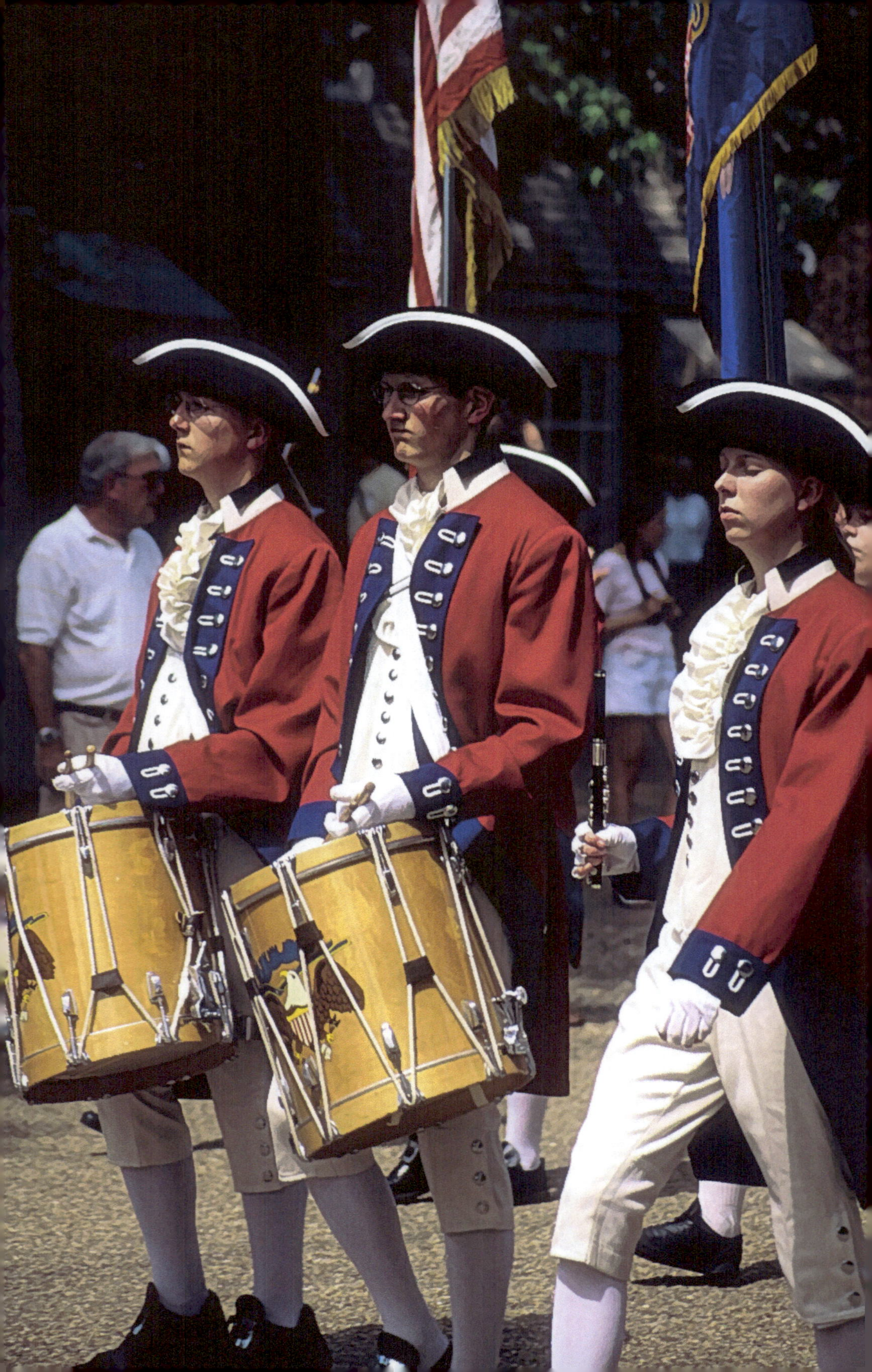

COLONIAL WILLIAMSBURG

Williamsburg was the capital city of colonial Virginia, the largest of the thirteen original American colonies.

Today, a 301-acre portion of Williamsburg stands as a living museum of that period, including hundreds of historically furnished buildings.

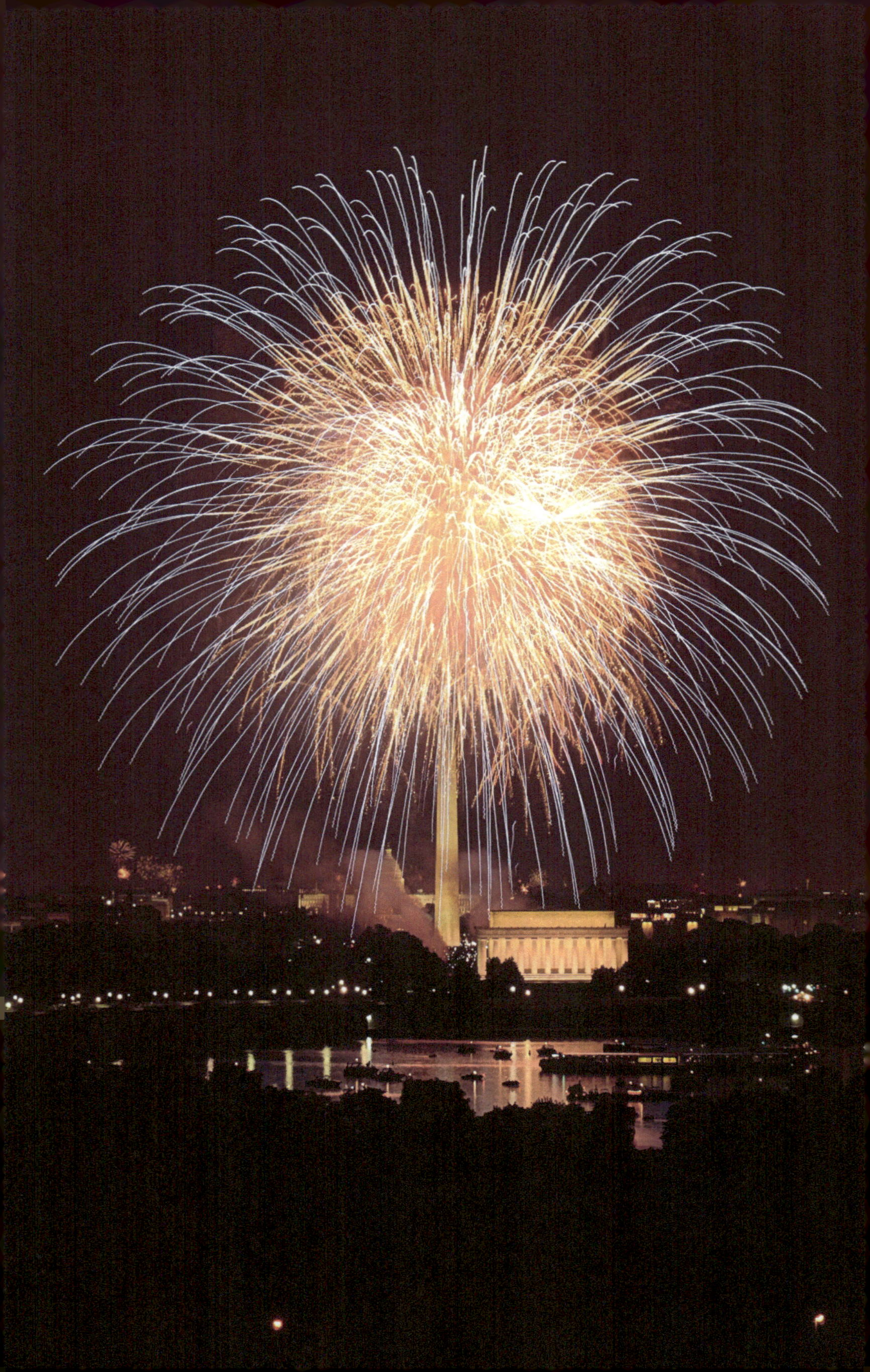

THE FOURTH OF JULY

The Continental Congress approved the final wording of the Declaration of Independence on July 4, 1776. But it wasn't until 1870 that Congress declared the Fourth of July to be a national holiday.

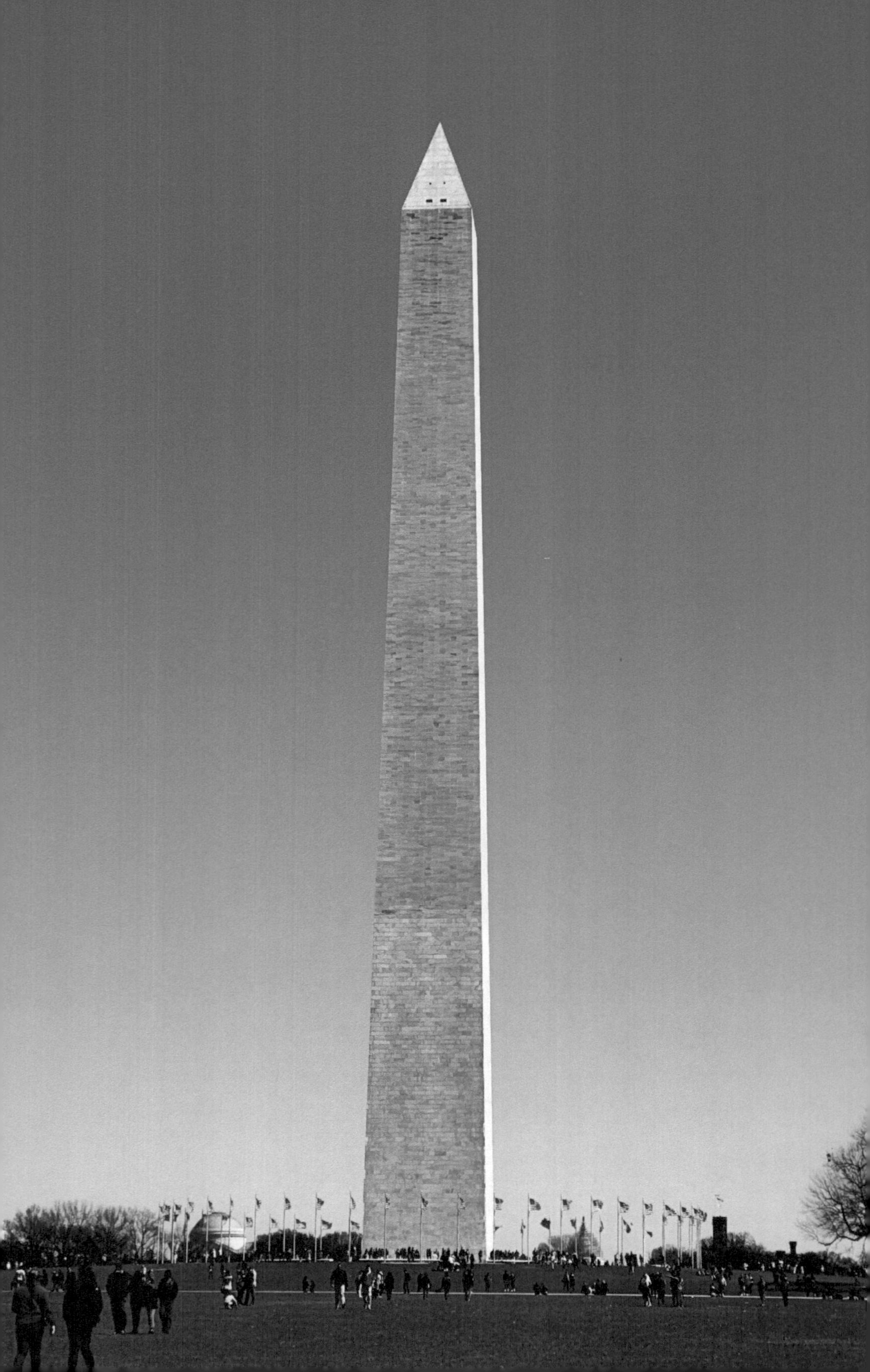

THE WASHINGTON MONUMENT

The Washington Monument stands on the National Mall in Washington, D.C. It was built to honor George Washington, commander-in-chief of the Continental Army and the first President of the United States.

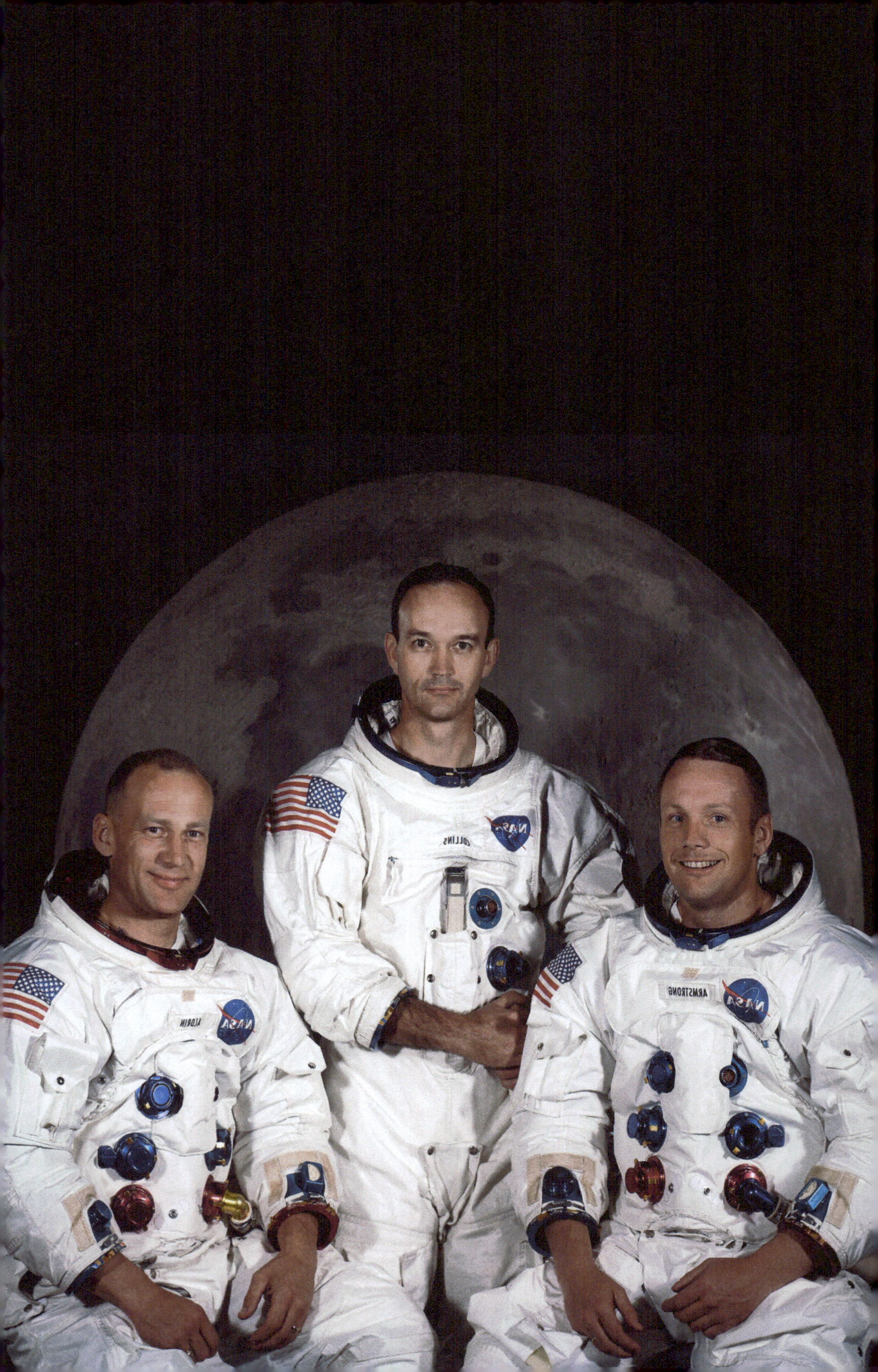

A MAN ON THE MOON

In 1961, President Kennedy pledged that America would put a man on the moon before the decade was out. That goal was achieved on July 20, 1969, when Apollo 11 commander Neil Armstrong stepped off the Lunar Module's ladder onto the surface of the moon.

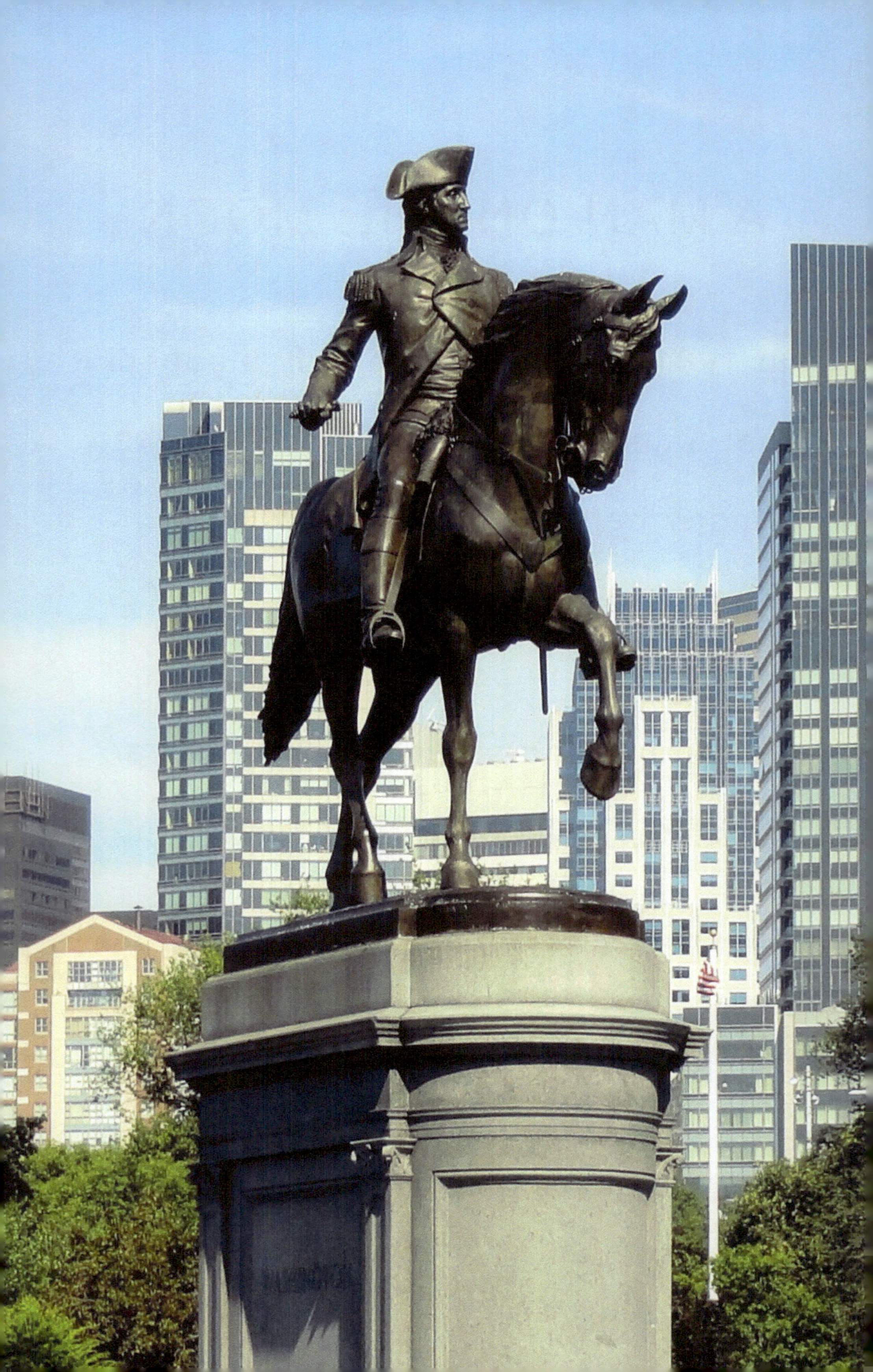

PAUL REVERE'S RIDE

Paul Revere's dramatic horseback ride on the night of April 18, 1775, warned Boston-area residents that the British were coming. Because of Revere's warning, the minutemen were ready the next morning on Lexington green for the historic battle that launched the American Revolution.

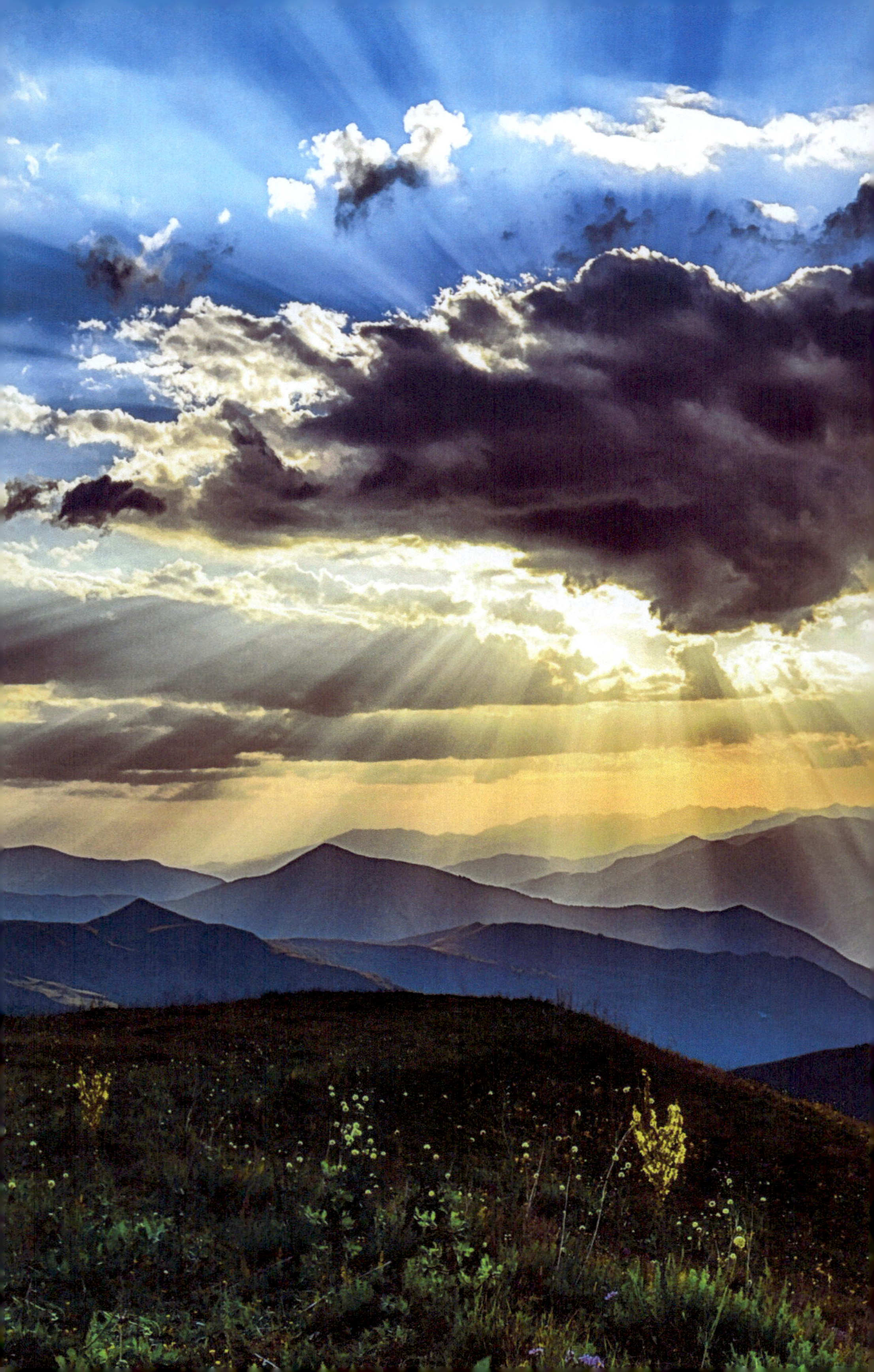

GOD BLESS AMERICA

♪ God bless America, land that I love

Stand beside her, and guide her,

Through the night

With the light from above.

From the mountains, to the prairies,

To the oceans white with foam

God bless America,

My home sweet home.

God bless America,

My home sweet home.

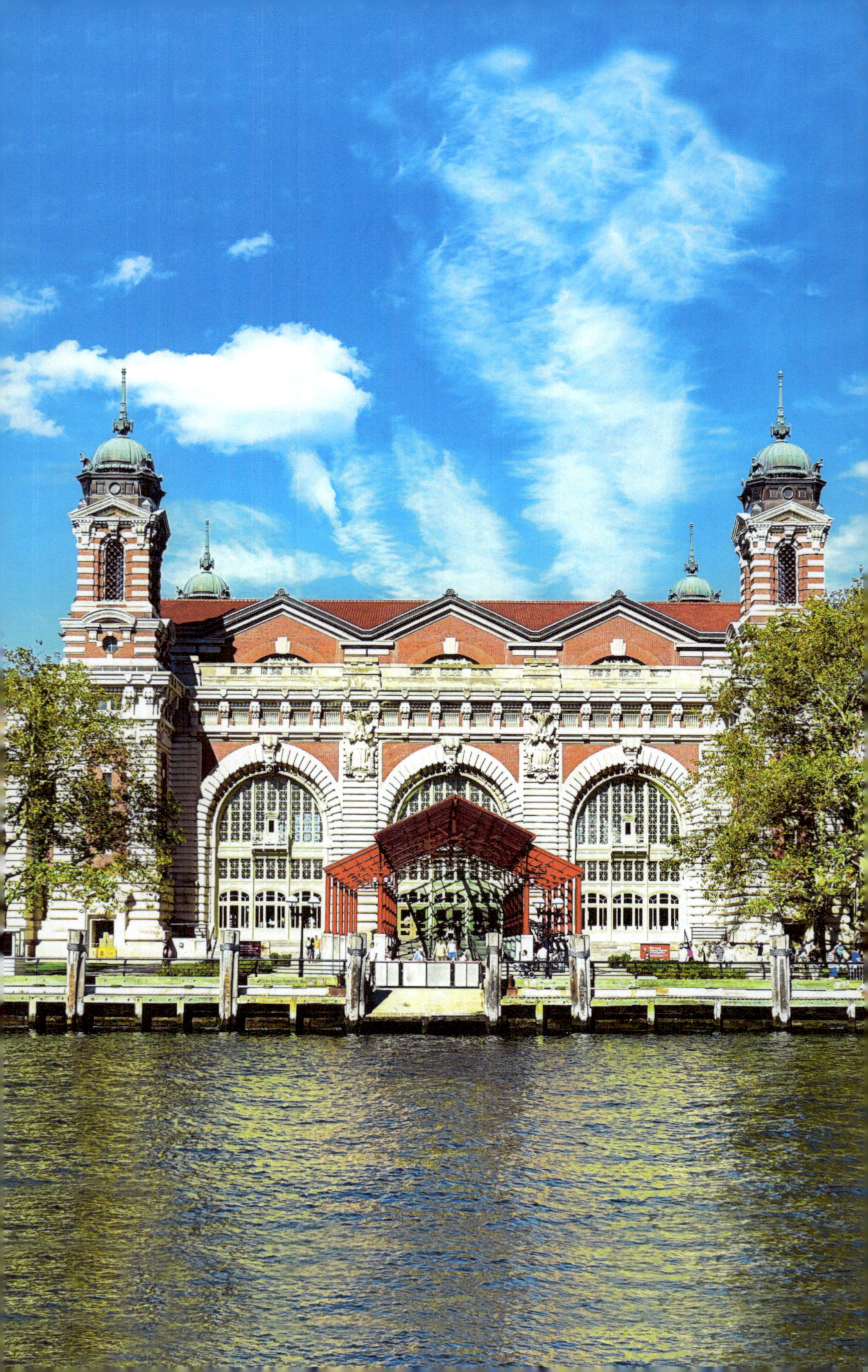

ELLIS ISLAND

Ellis Island was America's busiest immigrant inspection station from 1892 to 1954. Millions of newly arrived immigrants passed through its doors. Almost 40 percent of all current citizens have at least one ancestor who passed through Ellis Island when they arrived in America.

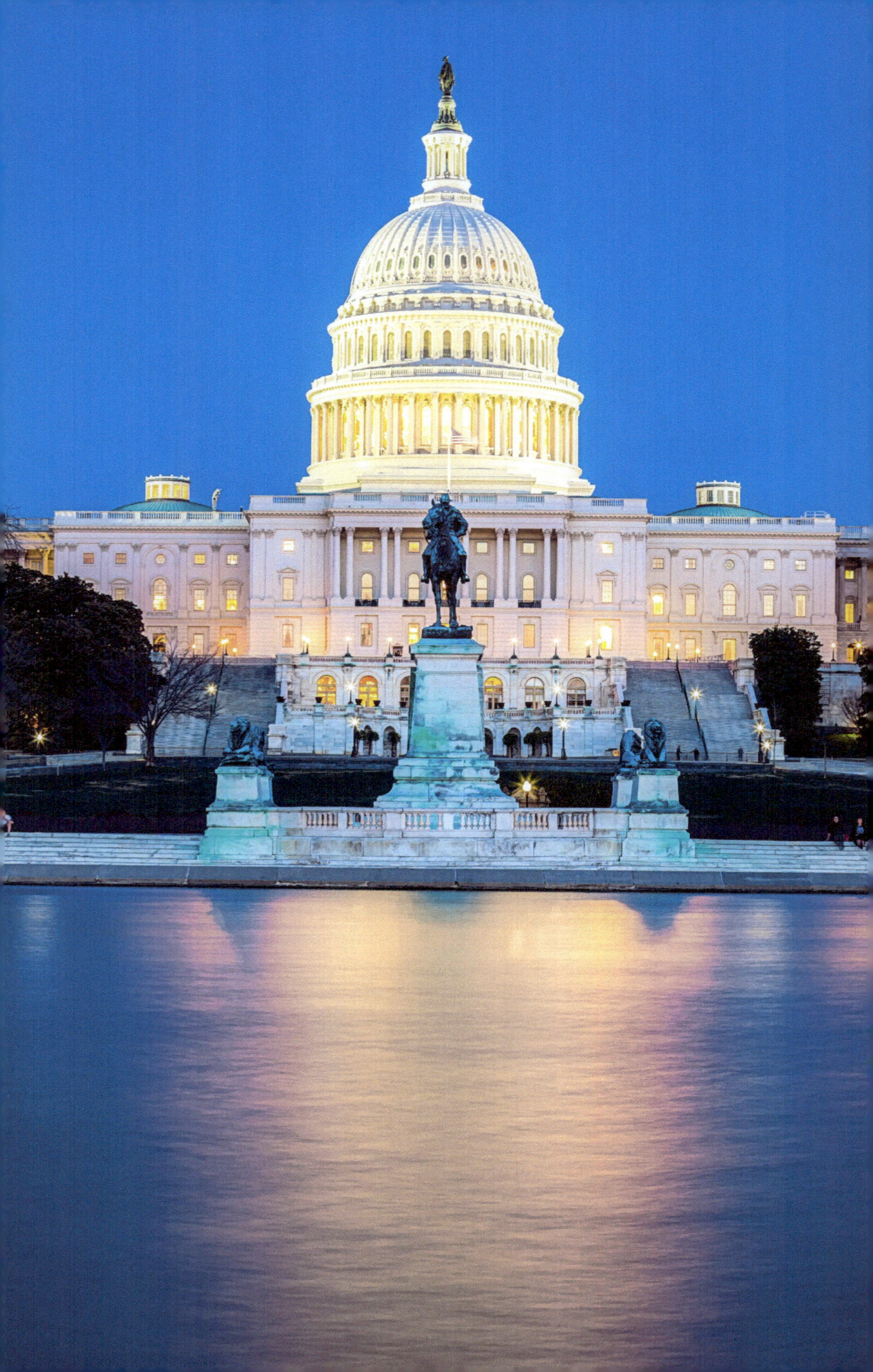

THE UNITED STATES CAPITOL

The United States Capitol in Washington, D.C., is the home of the United States Congress and the seat of the legislative branch of the United States government.

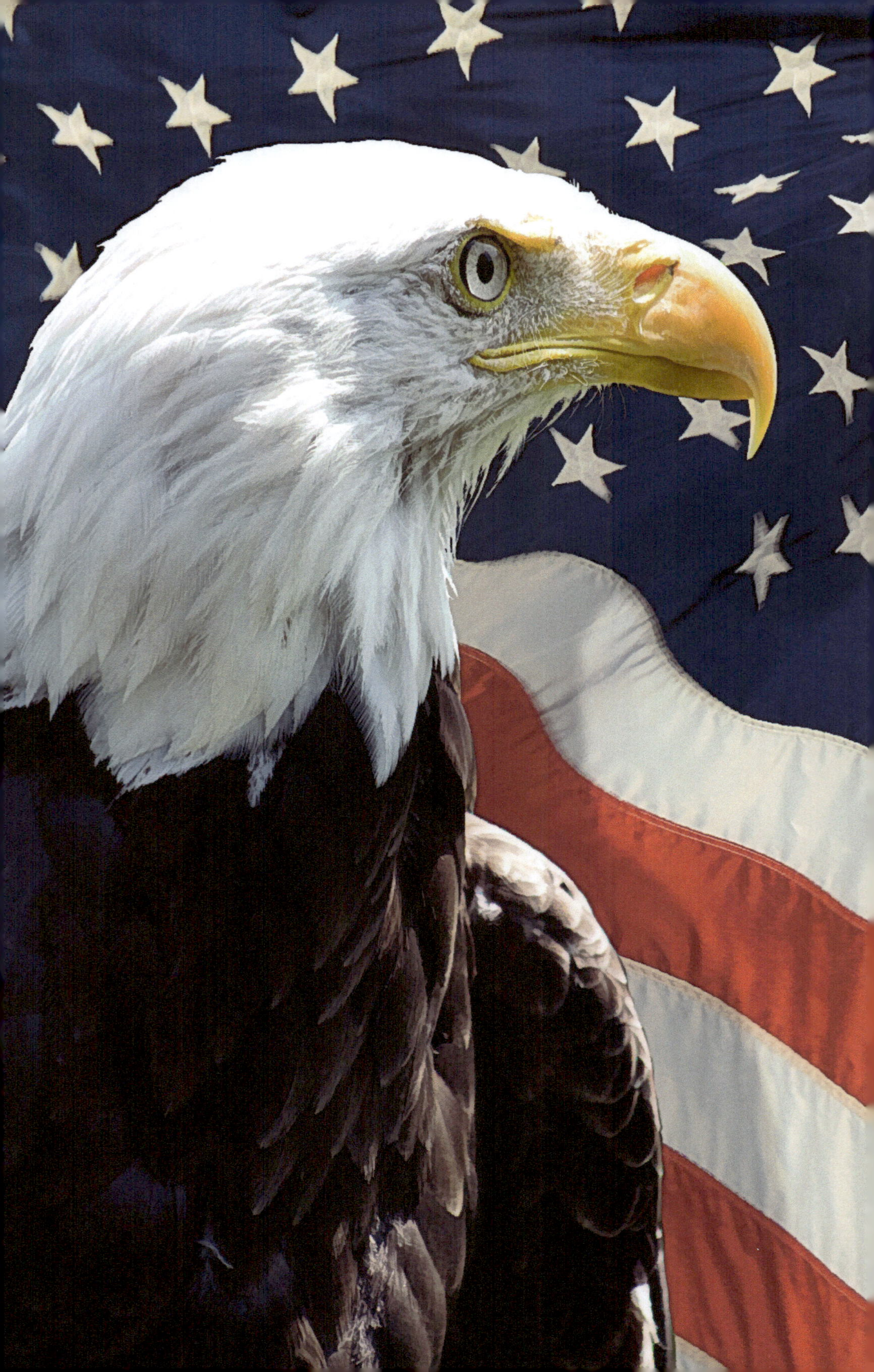

THE EAGLE

There is a legend that during one of the battles of the Revolutionary War, eagles took to the skies and began crying out. The patriots imagined that they were shrieking for freedom. In 1789, the eagle was designated as the national symbol of America.

www.ingramcontent.com/pod-product-compliance
Lightning Source LLC
Chambersburg PA
CBHW041808260726
48664CB00036B/1470